Who Will I Be? It's All Up To Me!

Written & Illustrated by

Dr. Maria Trent Corey

Copyright © 2021 Dr. Maria Trent Corey

ISBN: 979-8-7011-8123-4

All rights reserved. No part of this book may be reproduced, stored, or transmitted by any means—whether auditory, graphic, mechanical, or electronic—without written permission of both publisher and author, except in the case of brief excerpts used in critical articles and reviews. Unauthorized reproduction of any part of this work is illegal and is punishable by law.

To my son, Christopher –

You can be and do anything you put your mind to.

God has richly blessed you with many gifts and talents.

Shine your light on the world!

Love always,
Mommy

Your beliefs become your thoughts.
Your thoughts become your words.
Your words become your actions.
Your actions become your habits.
Your habits become your values.
Your values become your destiny.

– Mahatma Gandhi

Who Will I Be? It's All Up To Me!

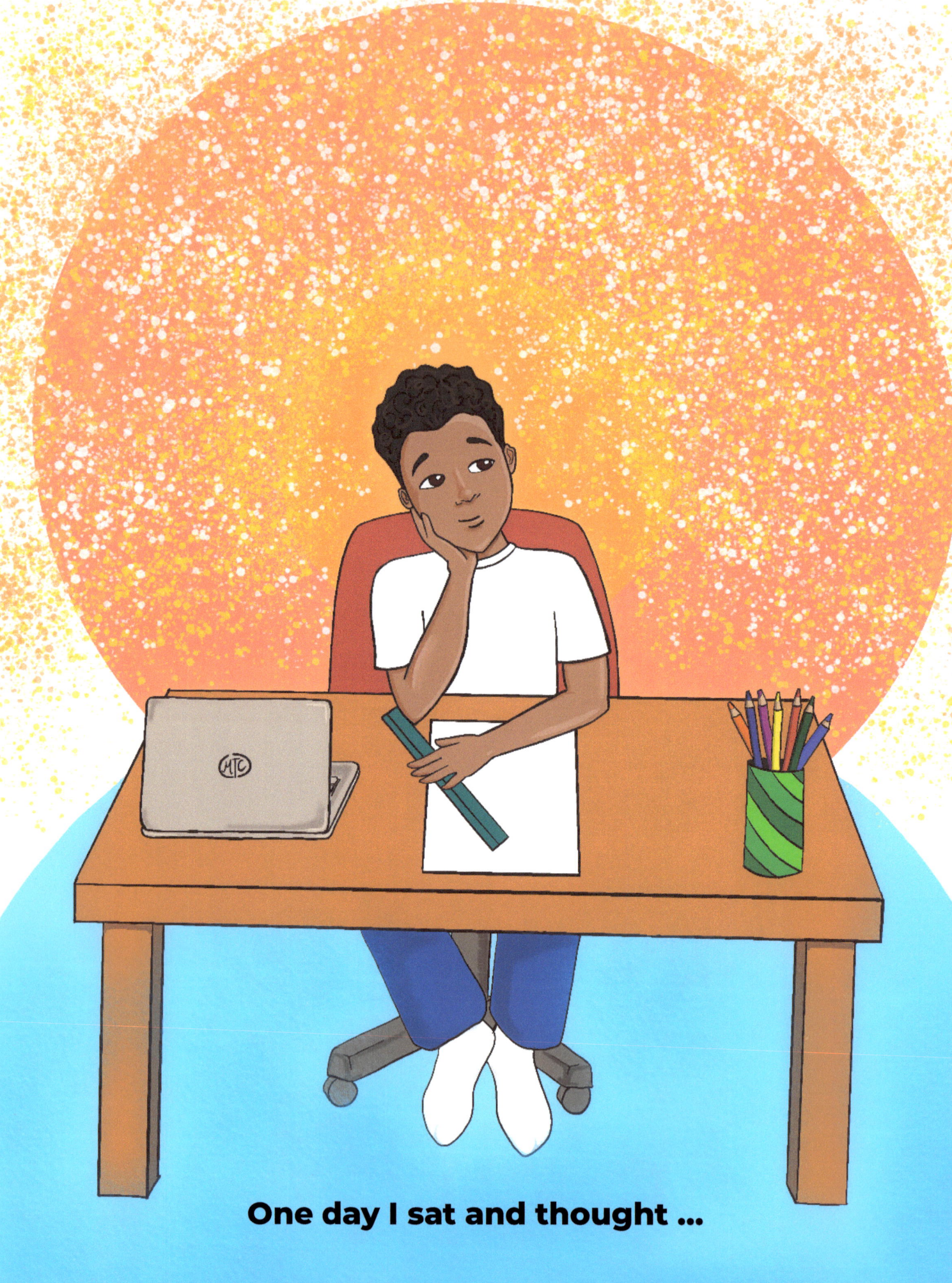

What does the future hold? Who will I be? How will I contribute to society?

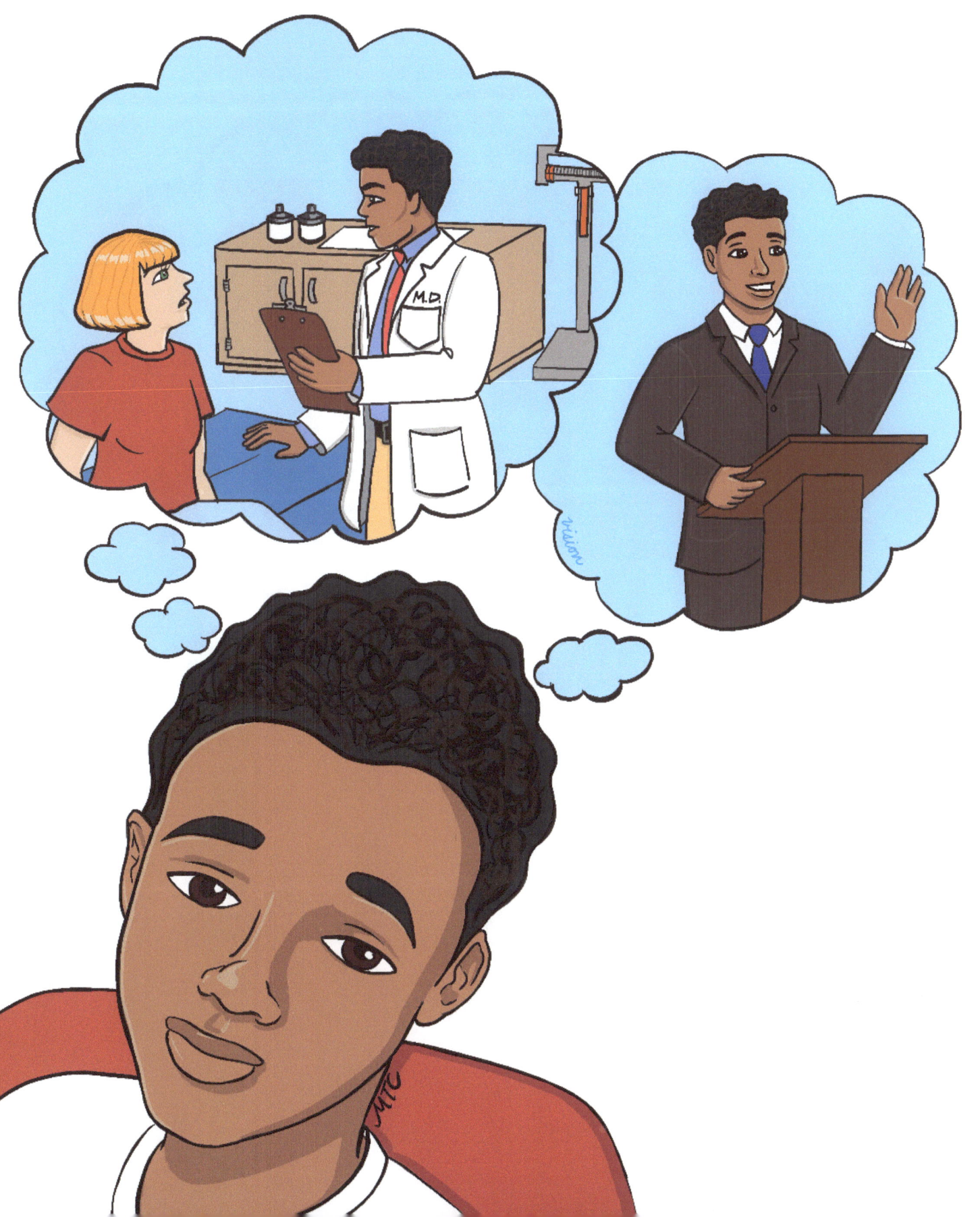

Will I be smart, strong, and wise?
Will I be kind or will I surprise?

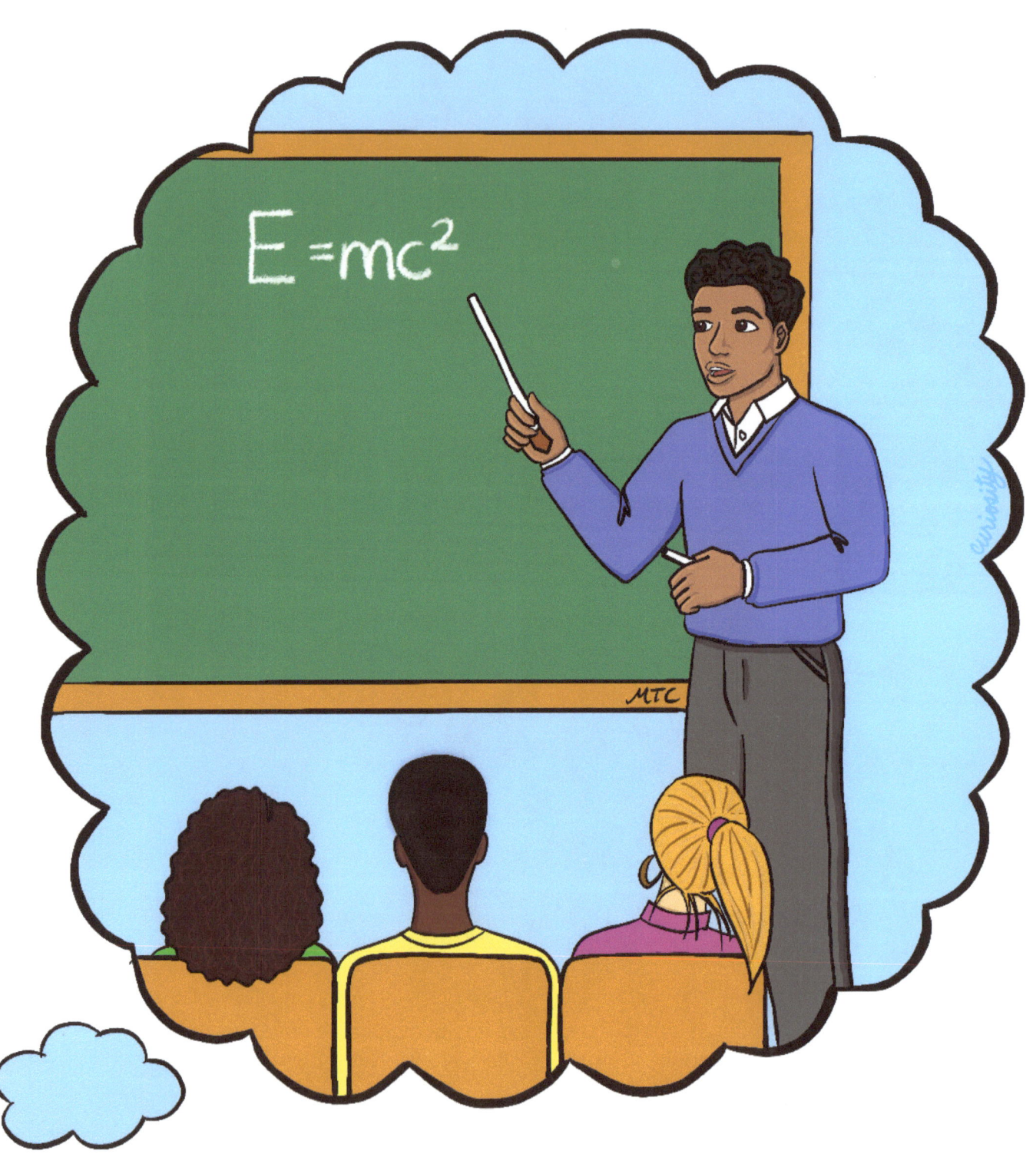

**Will I take care of a neighbor in need?
Will I be driven by more than greed?**

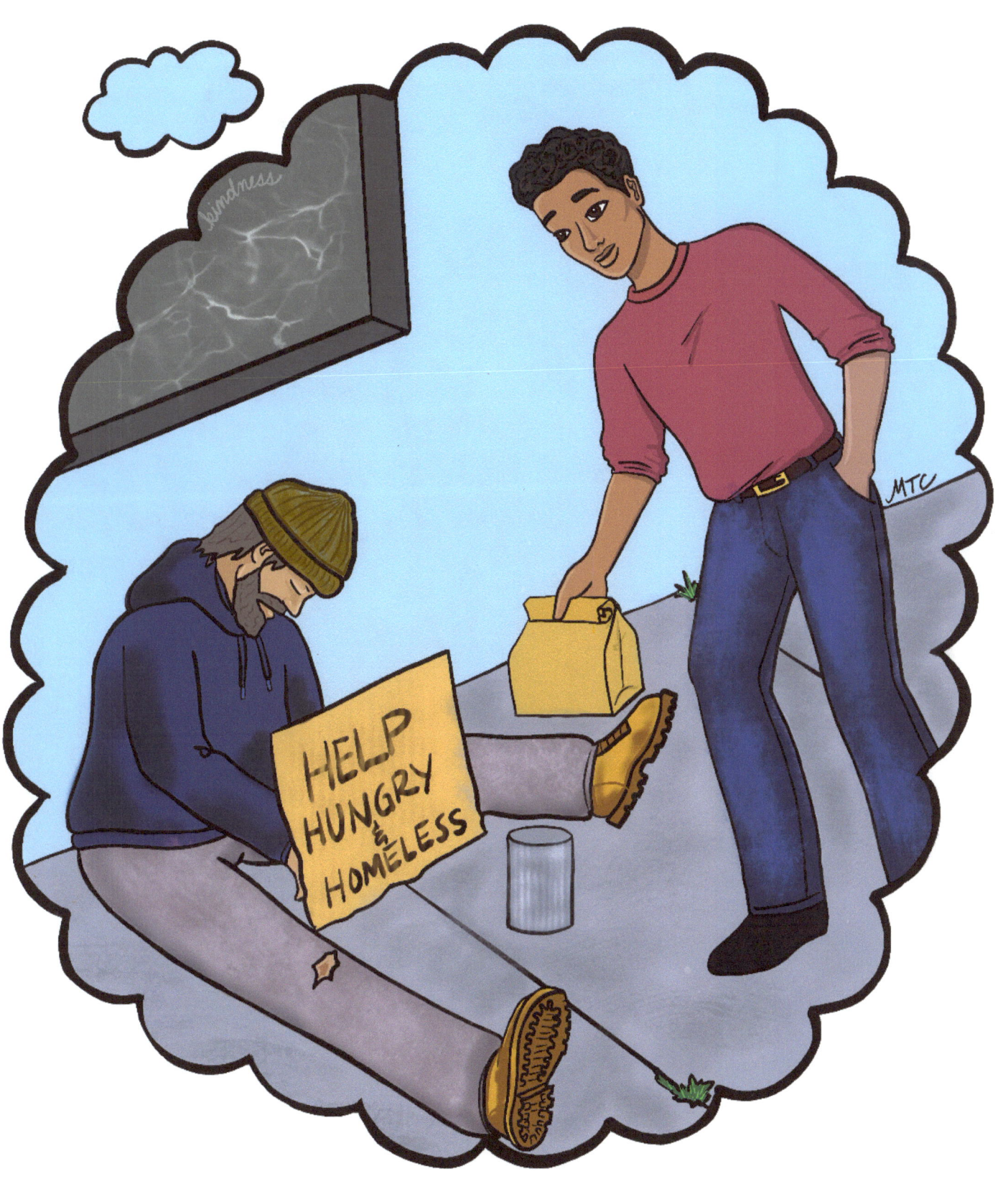

Will I speak up for those with no voice? Will I lead by example, make the right choice?

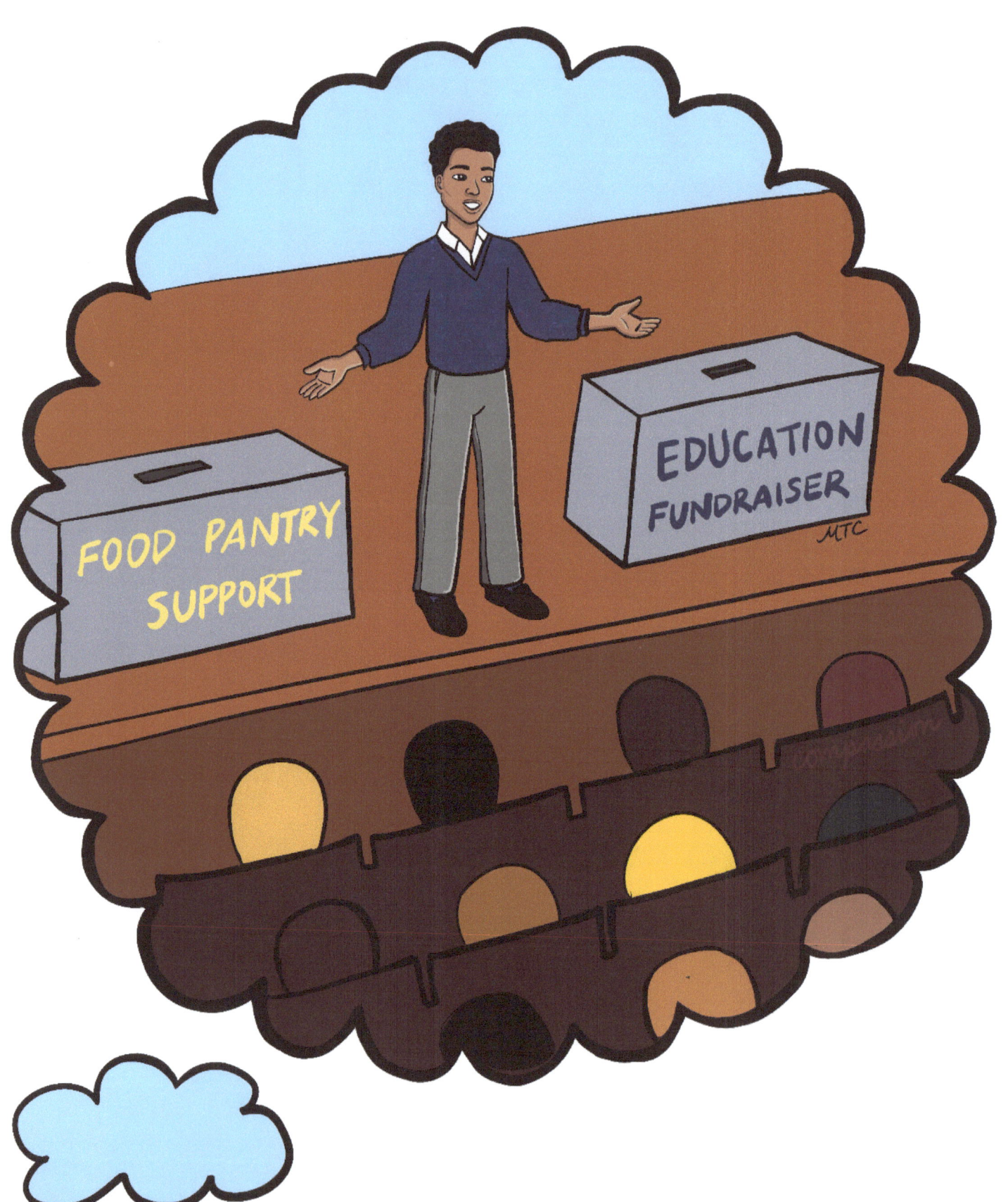

Will I stand up for what's right and good? Will I listen with patience until one's understood?

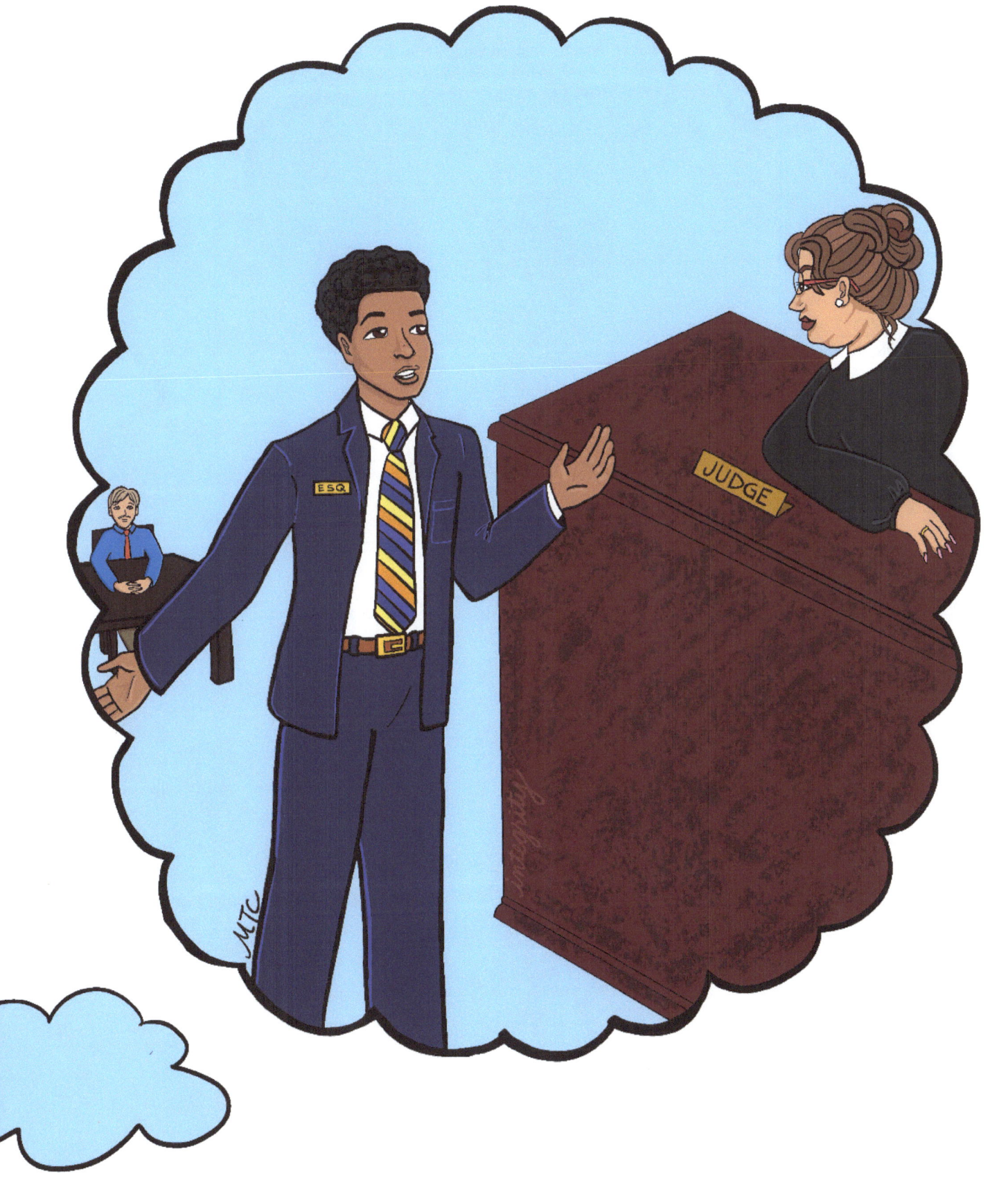

Will I bring people together in peace ... help stop arguments, make fighting cease?

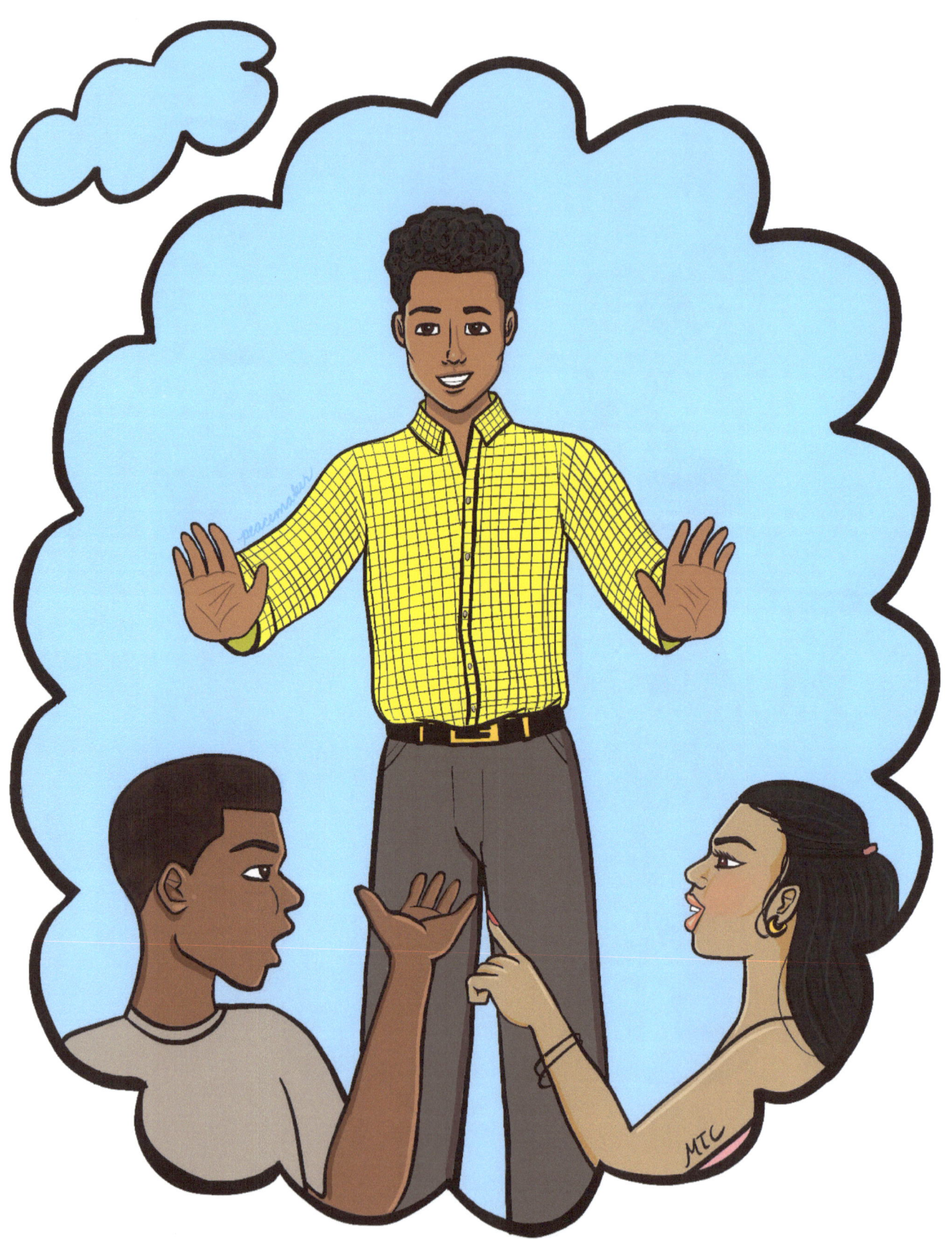

**Will I encourage others to do their best?
"Give your best try, no matter the test."**

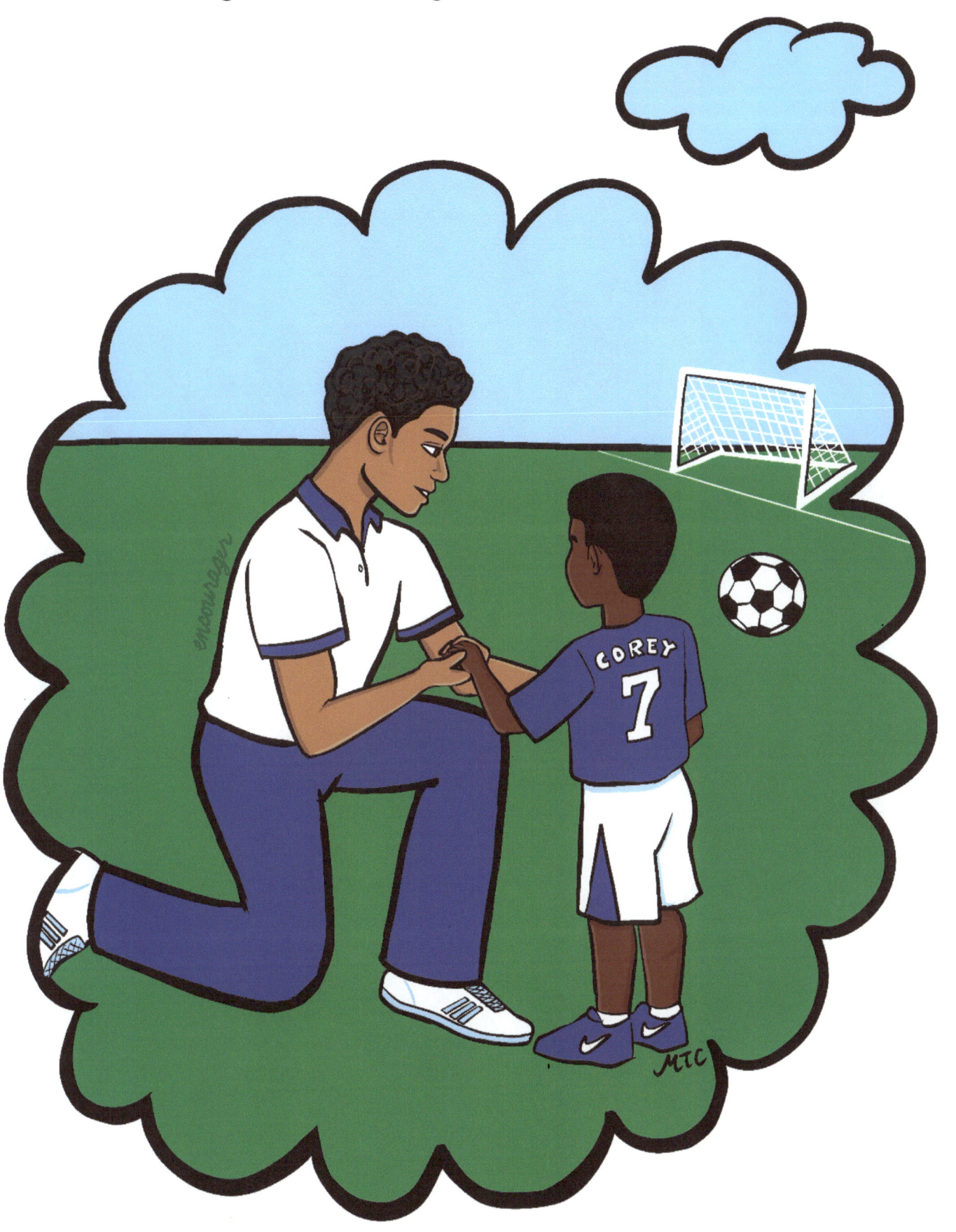

Will I be a light and let my gifts show? Will I share my talents with people I know?

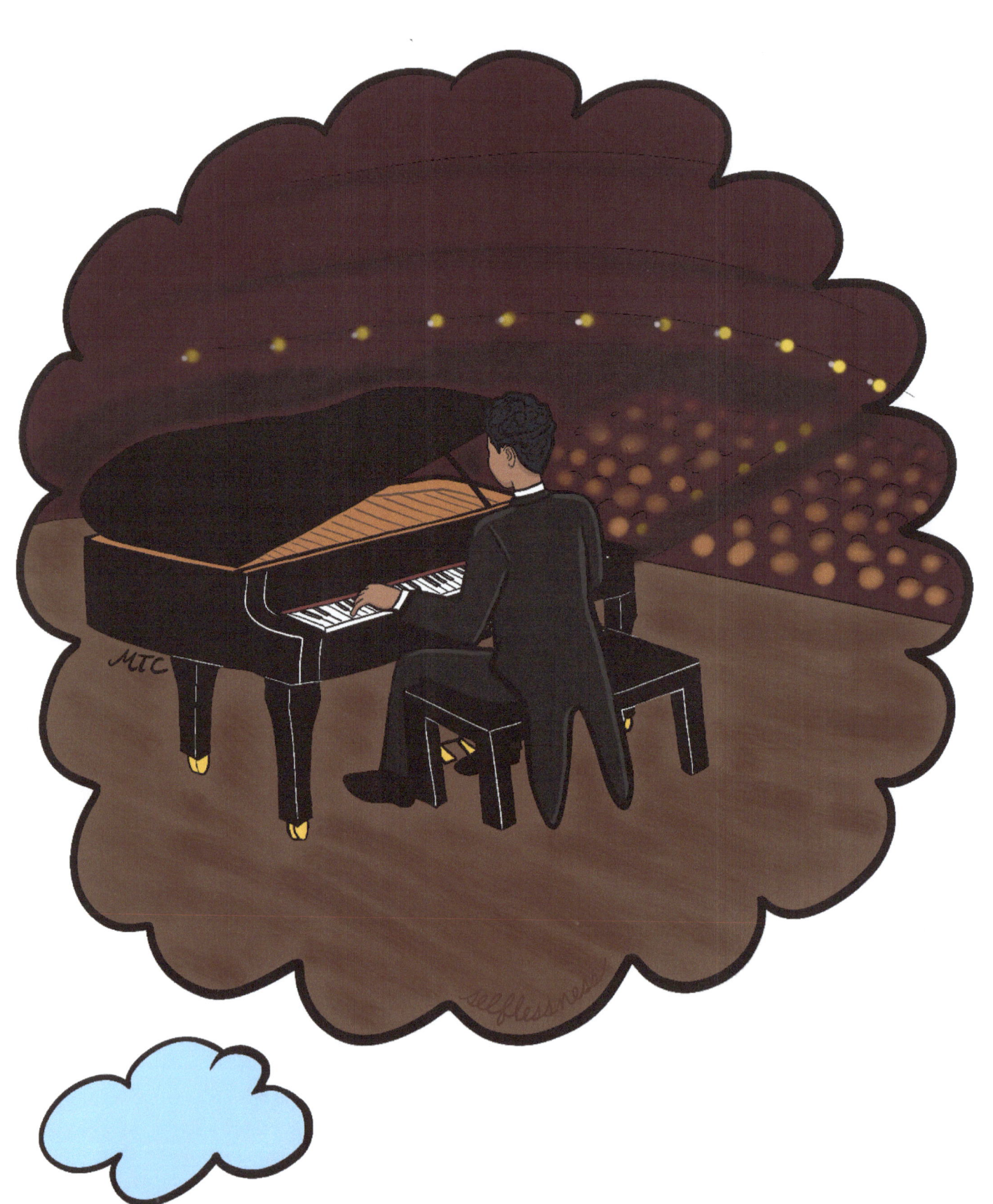

Will I accept those who think differently than me? Will I open my mind to see what they see?

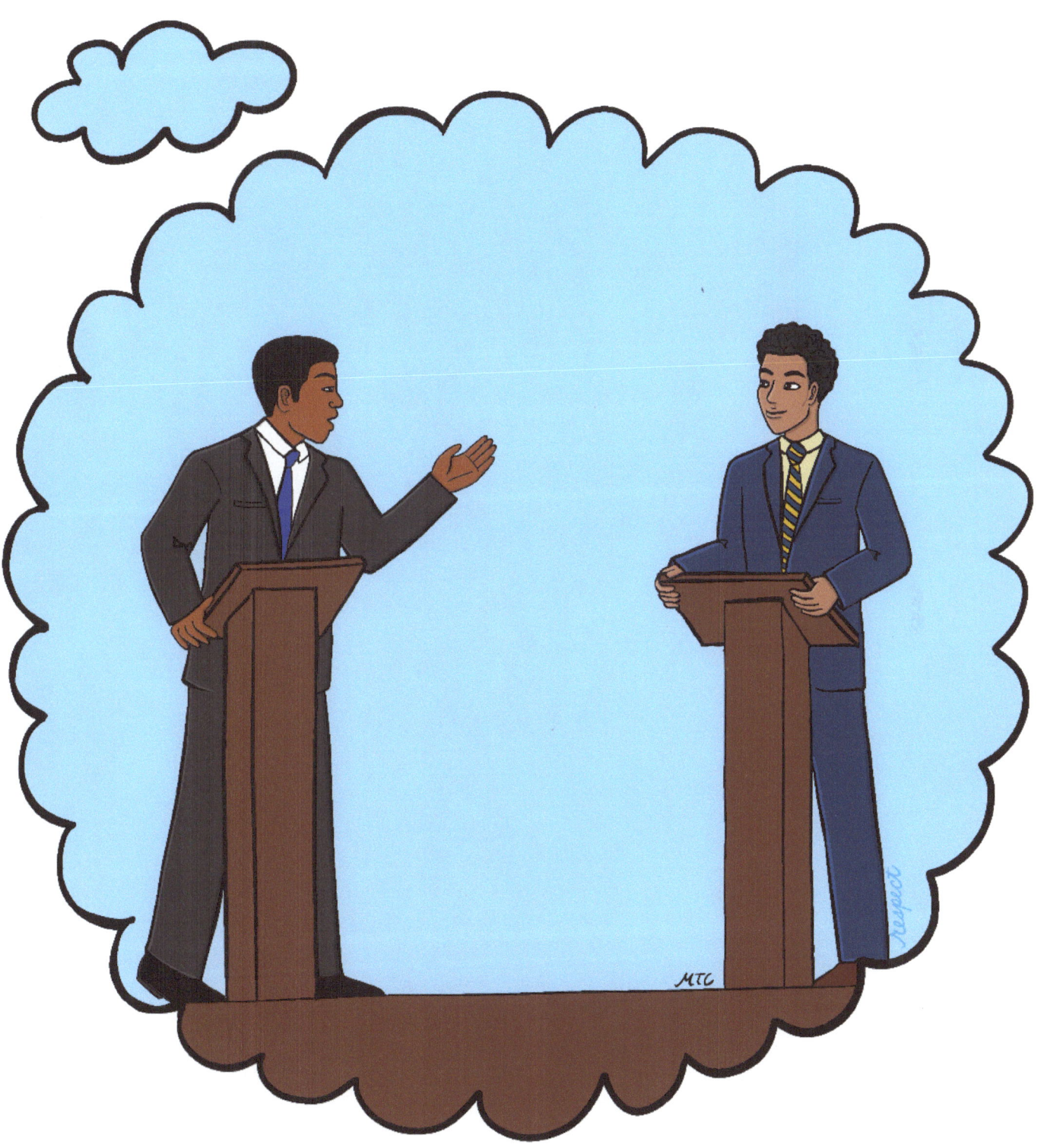

Will I learn from my neighbor, no matter their station? Everyone has something to offer... be patient.

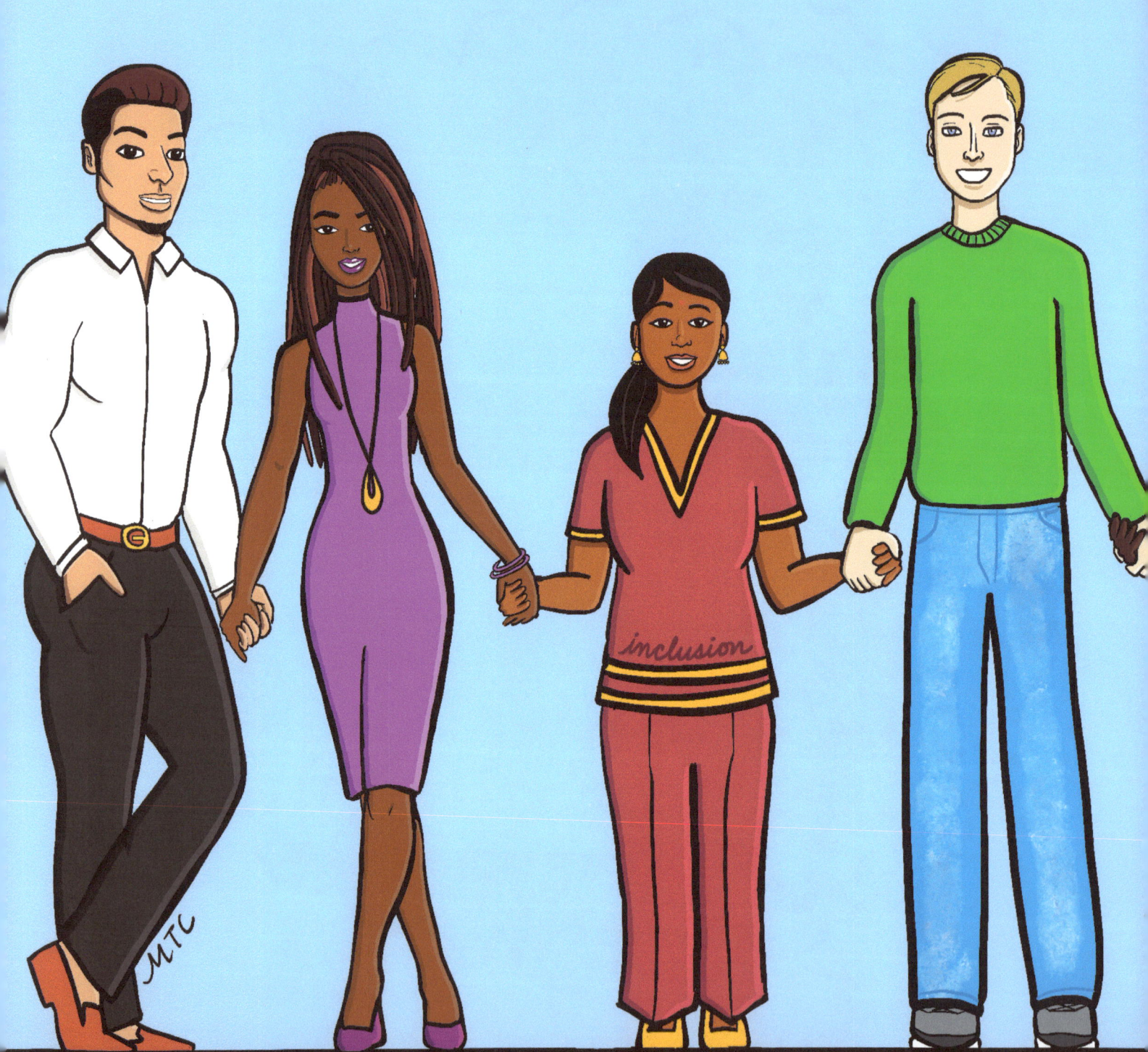

We all accomplish more with cooperation.

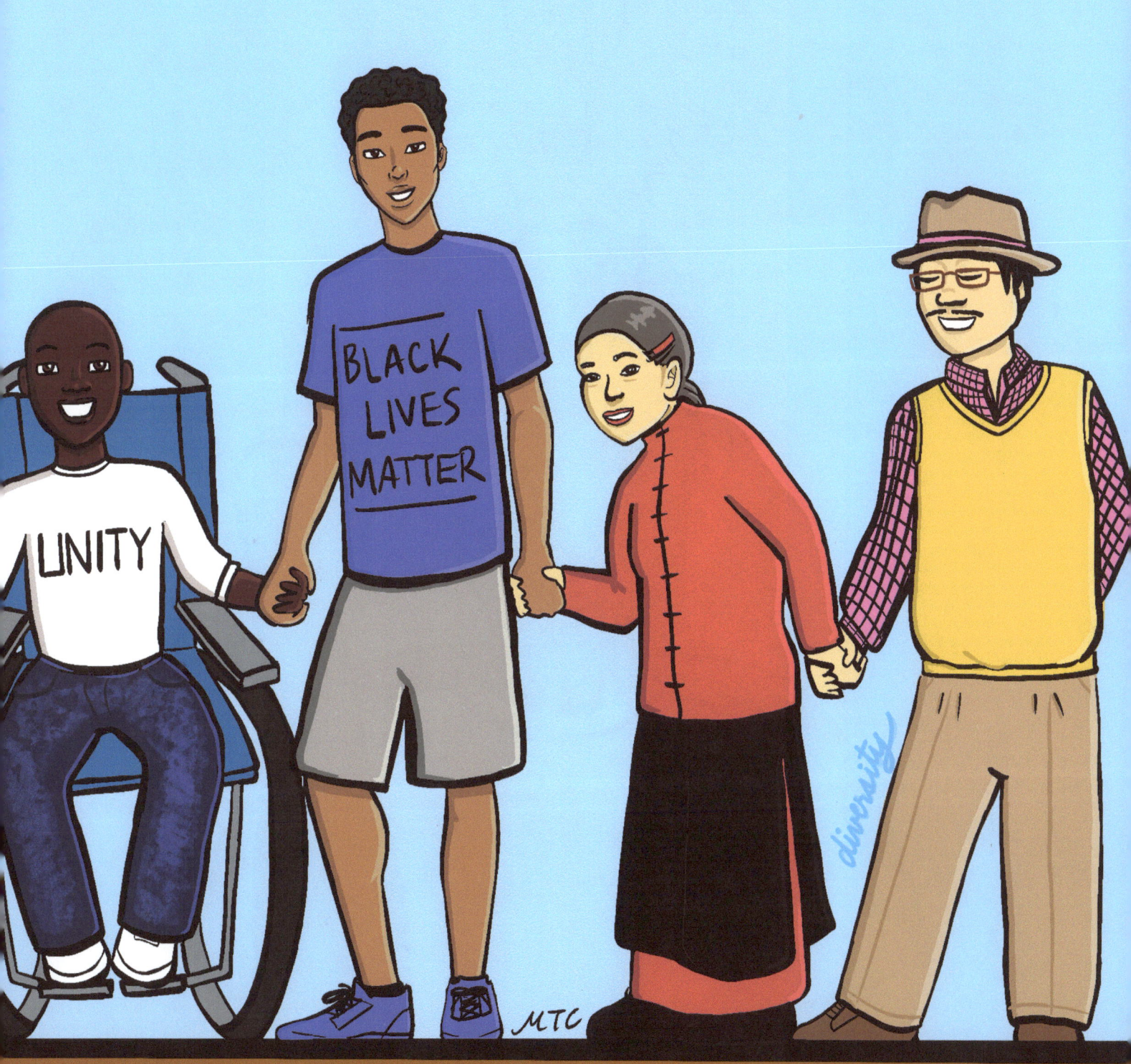

And that very day, it all became clear ...

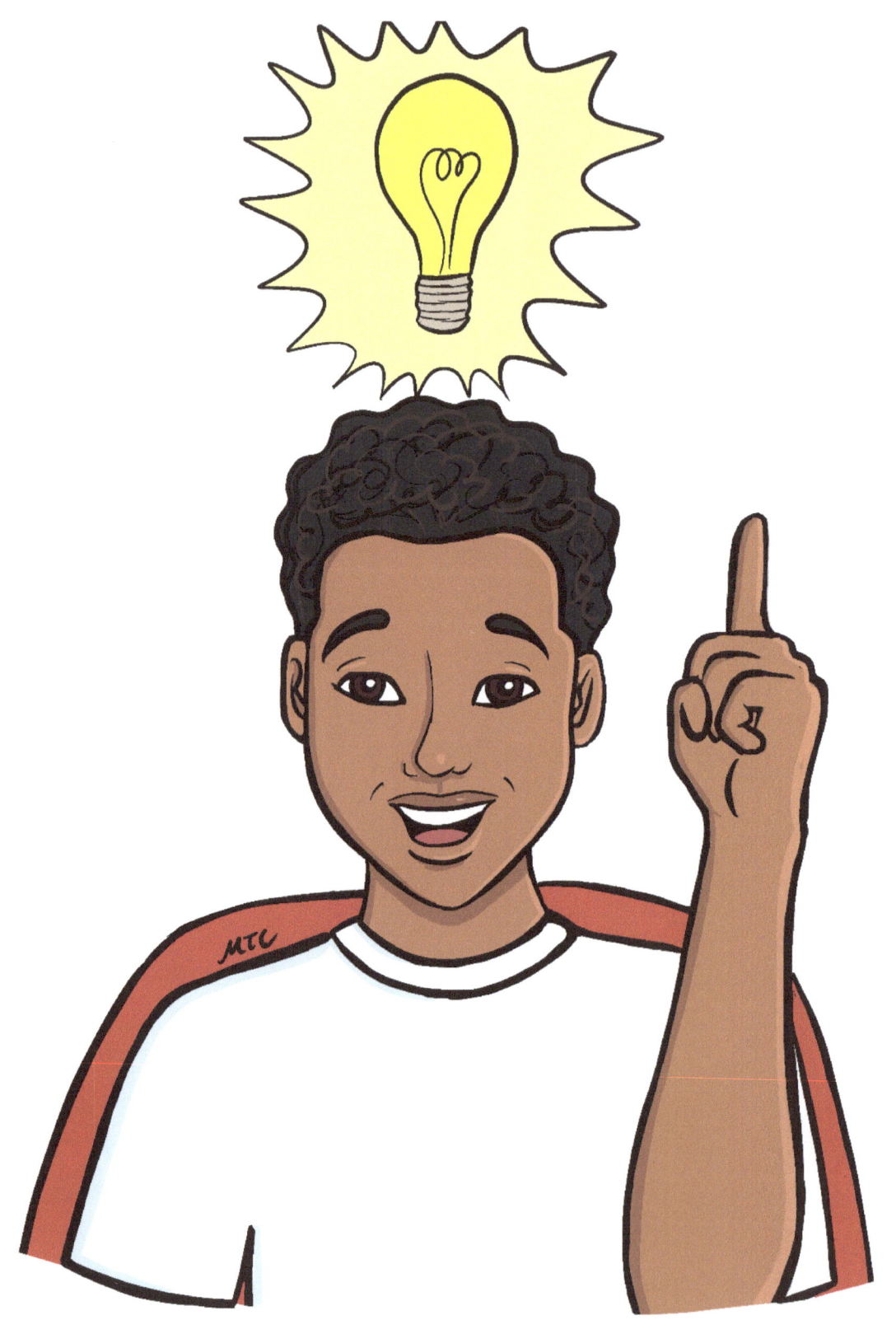

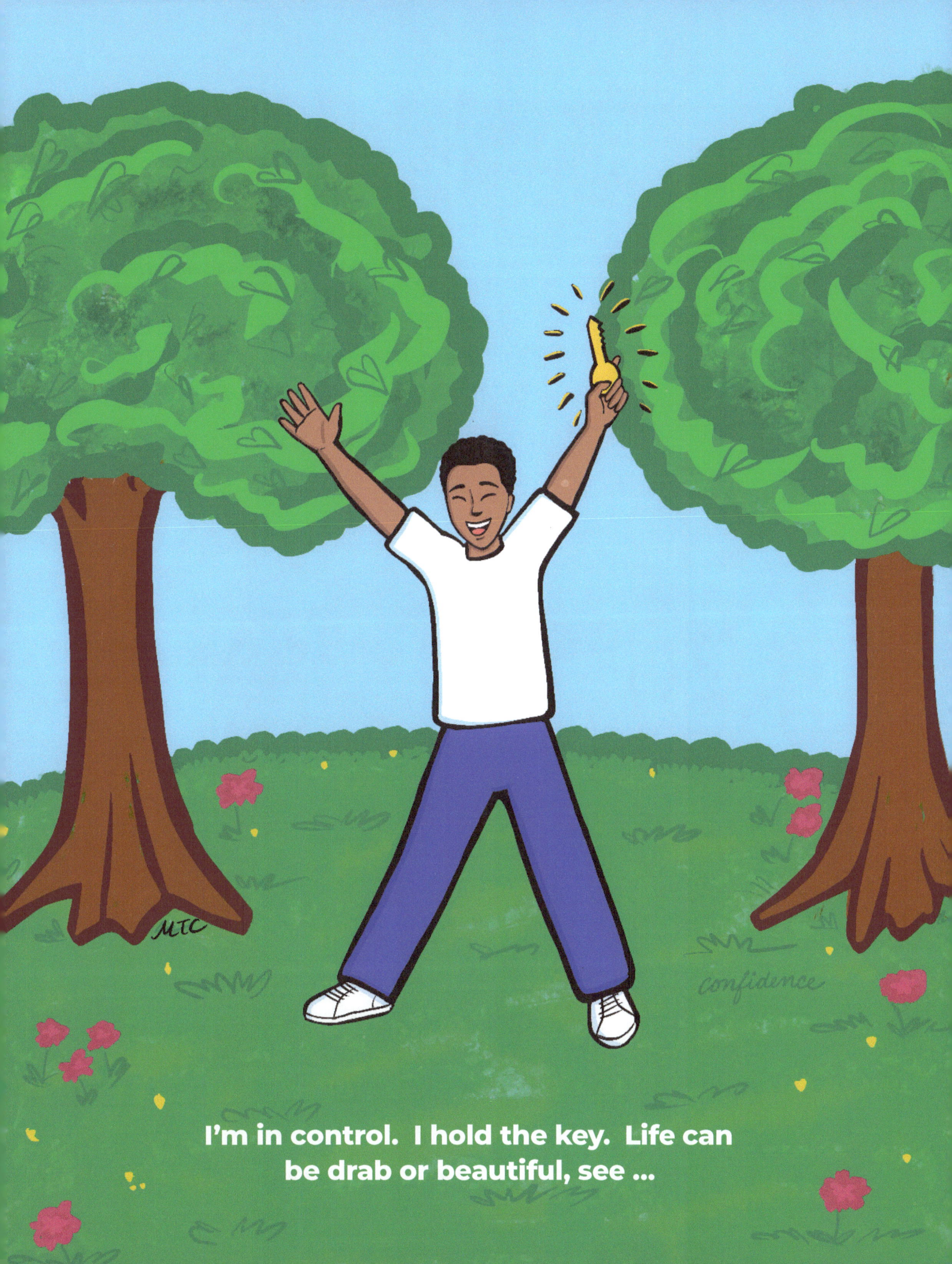

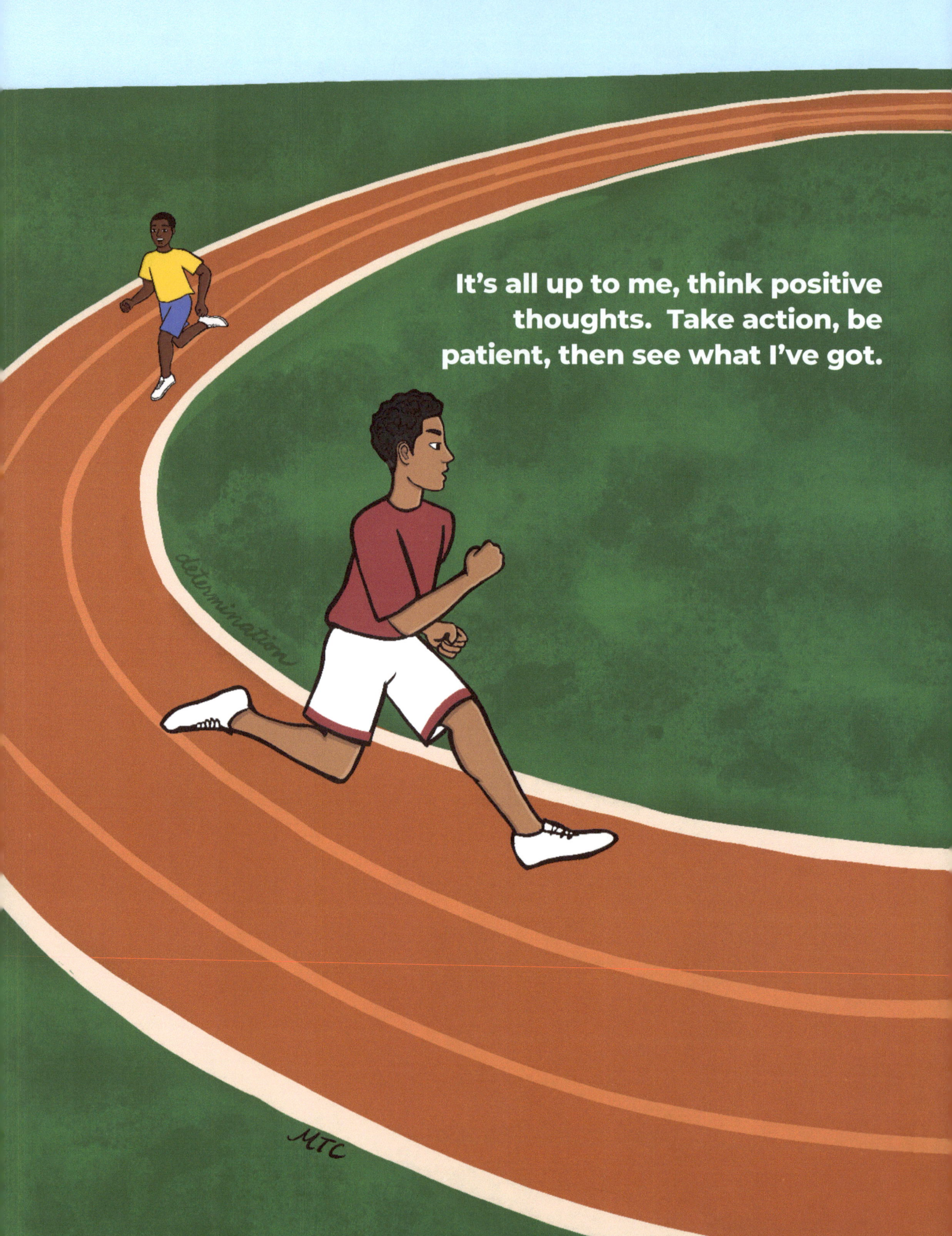

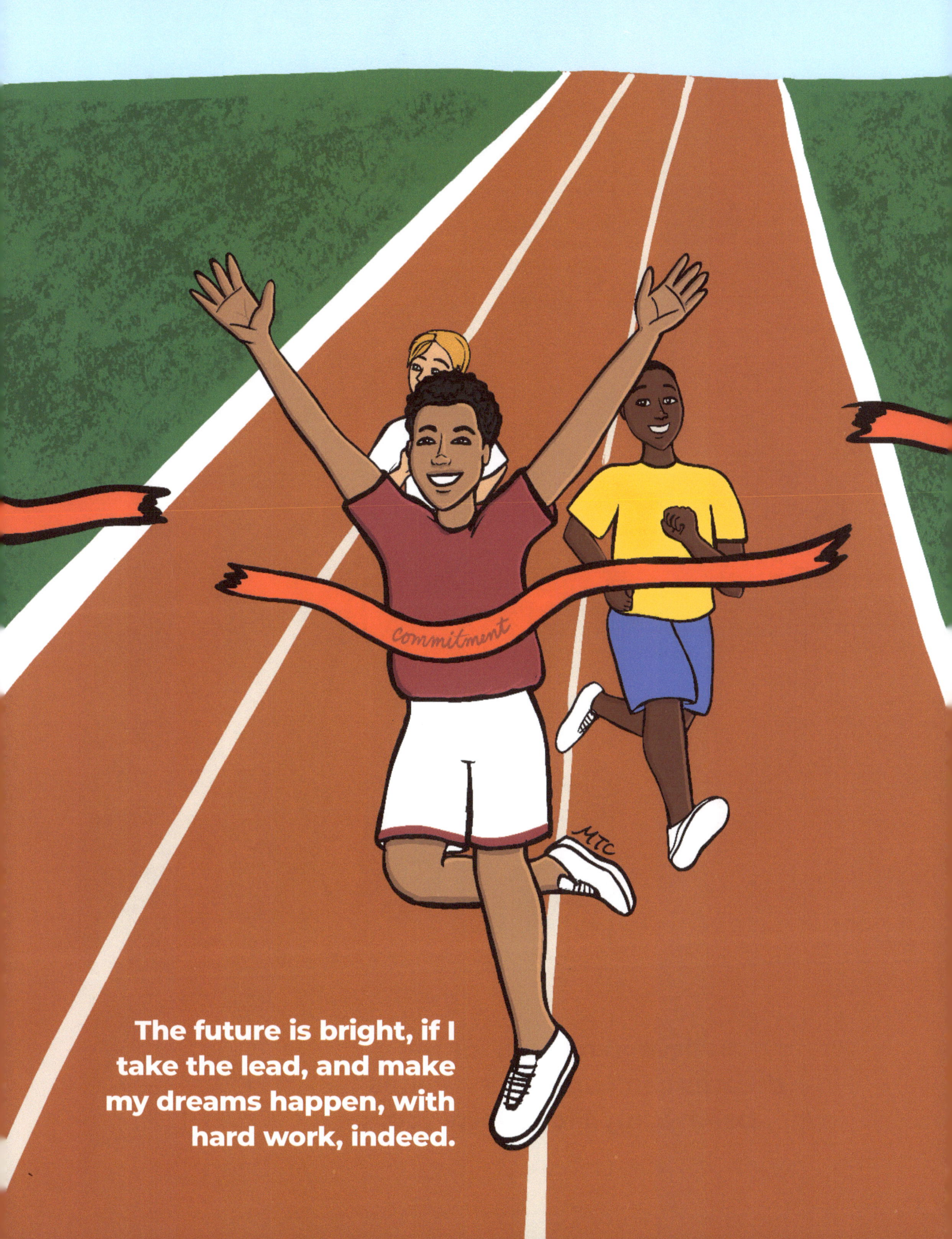

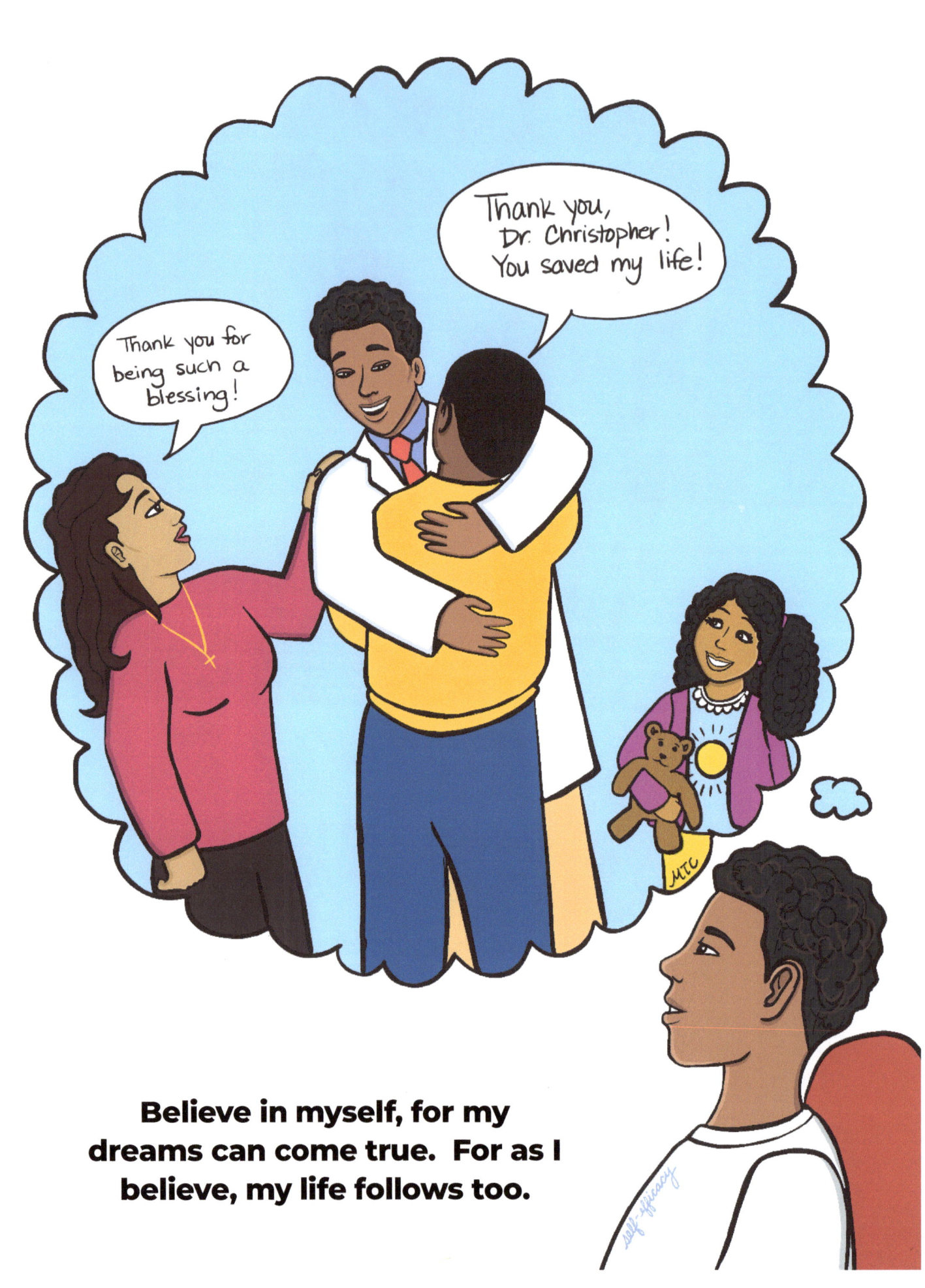

So, WHO WILL I BE?

Whomever I choose!

Dear parent or caregiver,

Thank you for purchasing this book for the special child in your life!

See if your child can find the positive values (hidden words) in the illustrations. After finding them, use the glossary to help define them for your child. Discuss with your child how they can incorporate these values into their daily lives to help others and reach their own goals!

All the best!

Dr. Corey

GLOSSARY

Vision	I can clearly imagine what I will be in the future.
Curiosity	I am excited to learn new things and find out about the world around me.
Kindness	I am friendly and I do good things for others.
Compassion	I care about other people and the things they go through.
Integrity	I am honest and I do what I know is right.
Peacemaker	I help people get along and see things in a common way.
Encourager	I help people believe that they can do their absolute best.
Selflessness	I think of other people, instead of only thinking about myself.
Respect	I know that all people are valuable and have something good in them.
Inclusion	I like to bring people together and not leave anyone out.
Diversity	I accept all people, no matter what they look like or where they come from.
Unity	We are all stronger when we work together and help each other.
Confidence	I believe in myself and in my abilities.
Determination	I have made up my mind to be successful and to reach my goal, no matter how difficult it may be.
Commitment	I have made up my mind to stay true to my purpose and to accomplish what I said I would.
Self-Efficacy	I know I can do anything I set my mind to do. I know I can handle any situation that comes my way.

www.ingramcontent.com/pod-product-compliance
Lightning Source LLC
Chambersburg PA
CBHW051838210526
45473CB00005B/1936